Meal Prep Cookbook:

50+ Quick and Easy Meal Prep Recipes for Weight Loss, Clean Eating and a Healthy Lifestyle.

Sarah Maddington

About Sarah Maddington

Sarah Maddington was born and raised in Manchester, UK. She is a Weight-Loss coach, Dietitian, Professional Chef and a mother of two. After finishing high school, she moved to London to pursue her dreams to study culinary.

In the past, Sarah was very overweight and suffered many health problems. She struggled with weight issues and found it difficult to maintain the balance between her career and her health.

It wasn't until after giving birth to her eldest daughter Sally, did she realise that she had to take her health more seriously if she wanted to become a role model for her children.
She lost 57 pounds in 6 months. Today, she wants to inspire beautiful people around the world to take control of the health so they can get back the life they deserve.

Table of Contents

Introduction

You may be wondering what meal prep is, and it's about to make your life ten times easier. You'll create a set menu, and then prepare your meals a head of time, which is perfect for the busy person. You'll need to schedule time to cook several meals, pack them, and then you can have them read to grab on the go. There are different types of meal prep planning, and we'll go over your two options in this chapter.

Long Term Prepping

This type of meal prep means you're planning three or more days in advance. You will need an afternoon to purchase all of the ingredients. Then you'll need to prep ad cook everything, and you'll have to have containers to keep them in. some people use resalable plastic bags, glass boxes, or plastic containers. This will take more time and effort, but the rewards are great. You don't have to cook for three to seven days, which frees up your schedule so that you can get more done.

Short Term Prepping

You'll be preparing for anything less than two days, which can be just organizing your breakfast for the next days. This will make it easier because you can just put your food in the toaster or oven and be done with it. Other people choose to marinate their meats for a day or two in advance. This will significantly reduce the time that you need to cook, but you'll still have to cook a few times a week. Some people choose to only prepare meals such as dinner, and other people prefer just to prepare their snacks in advance. Some people even meal prep without knowing. If you subconsciously pick up breakfast muffins in advance, this is a type of meal prepping! You may also pack leftovers to use for the next day's lunch, which is another type of short term meal prepping.

In this book you'll learn how too effectively meal plan and prep so that you free up even more time. You can use the tools in this book for short or long term meal prepping, depending on what time you have. This will free up time and help to reduce stress and anxiety.

So Why Do It?

This is a great way to feed yourself and your family healthy food every day without needing hours to cook. Time is short when you deal with your schedule, no less when you're dealing with other people too. Here are just a few benefits!

- **Saving Time:** Busy schedules are hard for everyone. When you choose what to eat at the last minute, it's likely not going to be healthy. Organizing your schedule becomes easier when you're not worried about food too.
- **Saving Money:** If you know what you're making for food, then you can plan your grocery shopping around sales. You can also buy in bulk, which will help to save you some extra cash.
- **Better Portions:** It's hard to measure how much you're eating if you're cooking last minute. Many people overeat on accident, but when you control your portions by making your food ahead of time, you'll know exactly how much you're eating each and every day. You won't have to worry about overeating, and you'll get all the nutrients you need!
- **Easy Schedule:** A more organized life means you have an easier schedule. Meal prepping frees hours every single day up for you to use for other things!
- **Healthier Meals:** Remember that fast food is often terrible for you. You'll get high sugar and high fat meals that won't do your body any

favors. When you plan in advance, you have healthier options made easier, which means you can stick to a healthier diet.

Meal Prepping Basics

Keep in mind that you need to aim for a healthy lifestyle when you use meal prepping, which is what it's mainly used for. This will help to keep your mental and physical health up, and it can help to reduce stress which leads to a healthier emotional health. Meal prepping is mean to be easy, and some people even find it to be fun! Here are some tips to help.

Be Simple

It's okay to not make anything too fancy, especially I you aren't used to meal prepping. Make sure that you pick out meals that are easy to make and that you enjoy. For example, smoothies are a quick meal you can prep too. Eventually you'll create your own recipes and tweak the ones you don't like too much to make a weekly meal plans that's completely your own.

Cook in Batches

Batch cooking means that you've set time aside to cook a large amount of different recipes in one sitting. So you'll make ten or more portions at a time, and then you can freeze them. It may seem like it's a lot of work, but it'll free up the time you need. Eventually, if you're using a deep freezer

Versatile Recipes

It's best to use versatile recipes. For example, maybe you're doing a turkey recipe that can be used or sandwiches or added to a soup. That recipe would have two different uses, and that is why it'd be a good recipe to prep in advance. Just make sure that you label it in a way that you know what it is, so that you can choose what you want to do with it! Mix and match recipes will be your best friend.

Fresh Ingredients

It's best to use fresh ingredients because you won't lose all the nutrients by freezing them. Just purchase fresh food, and use it as soon as possible. Making sure that you have nutrient dense ingredients is important to eating a healthier diet.

Keep a List

It's best to keep a list of everything that you have in your freezer or you may be at a loss for what you should take out of your freezer. You'll also want to create a list of the ingredients you have to work with when you're cooking, but you don't have to have a physical list. A list on your phone will usually work for what you need, and it's easier to add things to it too. By keeping a list, you won't have to go to the store twice, and you won't have to root around the freezer for your meals, trying to figure it out. Just make sure that you have two lists so you don't get them confused.

Don't Freeze Everything

There are some foods you just shouldn't freeze. Remember that not every food has to be frozen. There are some foods that can last at least two to three days in the fridge, and other foods will last two to three weeks in the freezer. The list of foods that can't be frozen is short, but you'll find it below. They'll taste different and have a different texture when thawed, which is best to be avoided.

- Cooked Eggs
- Cooked Pasta
- Cheese or Crumb Toppings
- Sauces, Milk Based
- Mayonnaise
- Salad Dressing

- Fried Foods
- Raw Vegetables, Including Celery, Lettuce & Cabbage

The Right Containers

If you're meal prepping, then you're going to need containers to keep it in. of course, there are a few do's and don'ts that you'll want to keep track of! The right containers will make a huge difference in the quality of your meals. You don't want to heat up a frost bitten meal, since it won't taste the same. It can even cause you to get sick, so make sure you have the right containers for the job.

Microwave, Dishwasher & Freezer Safe

It's important that you make sure that your containers will live through the meal prepping cycle. It needs to be able to deal with the cold of the freezer and the heat of the microwave, and no one wants to have to wash all of their dishes by hand. These types of containers may cost a little more, but by purchasing the right containers, they'll have a longer shelf life in your home.

Stack Them!

This is especially important if you have a small freezer or kitchen, since having stackable dishes will help you to manage your space. You'll want dishes that can stack on top of each other even if they're full to save space. Most people just find dishes that are stackable if they're empty, which only helps when they aren't being used.

Leak Proof

If a container isn't made properly, then you'll find that they leak through the lid. You should have containers that can be flipped upside down without leaking, which will make them perfect to take on the go. Once again, this will be more expensive, but they'll last longer and do better or your busy lifestyle. Nothing will ruin your appetite more than opening your bag to find your food has leaked over everything. If you aren't sure about the quality of your container, fill it with water, seal it and flip it upside down to check for leaks.

The Material

Even if you're just getting plastic, the type of plastic you get is important. There are cheap manufacturers that will make their dishes out of plastic that's easily damaged. This means you have maybe three to six months before you'd need to replace them. Investing in a higher quality plastic or glass container will be the better option since they'll last you three to five years despite their price tag. Some containers can even last over ten years if you keep them properly.

Your First Meal Prep Day

It's time to choose the day for meal prepping, which most people choose Sunday. Saturday and Sunday is popular because it's often a person's day off, but many people will choose Sunday since there are often less activities going on. If your time on your days off is limited, then get a slow cooker or an Instant Pot to help you. You'll need a long morning, or afternoon, to complete everything. In this chapter, you'll get an idea of what a meal prepping day looks like.

Step 1: Plan Your Meals

Figure out the meals that you'll want to prep, and then figure out what you need to make in advance. For example, if you want pancakes, then determine how many days you want to eat pancakes. You don't want to make too much or it'll go bad, but too little and you'll need to cook again too soon. Next, pick some alternatives for the other days, and then figure out the ingredients you'll need to buy. Write it down, and make a shopping list for everything you'll neeed.

Step 2: Go Shopping

Most people prefer to do this on the same day, but you can make your shopping list and shop in advance if you don't have enough time to set aside at once. It's best to buy bulk deals if you want to save money, and try to stick to your shopping list so that you don't stray to aisles that are full of unhealthy food.

Step 3: Start Organizing

Having an organized kitchen will make meal prepping a lot easier. If you're meal prepping the same day, most everything can be stored on the counter or in the fridge, but it gets more complicated if you're planning for another day. If you're meal prepping the next day, keep your meat in the fridge. If it'll be a few days, you'll need to decide if it's worth putting it in the freezer. If you got your meat on sale, perhaps marked down because it's old, then you may want to put it in the freezer so it doesn't go bad. This means you'll need to give it time to thaw before cooking though.

Step 3: Get Ready to Cook

Prepare all of your ingredients by measuring them out. This is option, of course. However, if you don't pre-measure everything it will take more time to actually cook your meals. Though, you will want to cut, slice and measure your meat. You'll also need to marinate any of your meats in advance. You may want to chop the vegetables after washing them if you can too. Just make sure that you're careful with browning.

With certain recipes, browning won't be a problem, but with others it can make a large difference on how your food ends up tasting. If you're doing a soup, some browning won't make a different. You can also spray water and lemon juice over your cut vegetables to keep them from browning. Many people prefer to submerge their cut vegetables in this mixture, but this can cause certain vegetables such as squash to become water logged, which will also change the flavor and texture of your food.

Step 4: Start Cooking

This is the easiest part! If you're using a slow cooker or instant pot, you can usually just throw it in and forget it. However, traditional cooking means you'll need to prepare your dishes by following the recipes, keeping the cooking time in mind. Some people prefer to double a small batch recipe, but there are many large batch recipes you can use in this book. Most people will not spend more than an hour or two cooking, depending on the recipes that you're making.

Step 6: Prepare Toppings

This means you'll need to prepare your dressing and sauces. Just remember that milk based sauces and salad dressings or casserole toppings do not do well in the freezer. You'll only want to meal prep this if you're going to keep in the fridge for a few days. You'll be able to take this step to create sides too, which take about fifteen to twenty minutes depending on the recipe. Store them separately than the rest of your meal!

Step 7: Package it All Together

While it can be best to keep certain sides and toppings separate than your actual food, you can still put them in the same container depending on the dividers. Divide your portions properly and then store them in either the freezer or fridge. With bigger portions, one large container to two boxes usually work best. You should also keep wet foods and dry foods stored separately until it's time to eat.

Tips & Tricks for Success

Meal prepping is great to save you time and eat healthy, but you may still be a little worried about prepping all of your meals in advance. Here are some tips and tricks to make it even easier!

Create a Cookbook

No one likes every recipe, so you'll want to keep a scrapbook or cookbook of your favorite recipes. Make it where you can jot down any alterations that you'd like to make for a dish that you've already tried, and you'll enjoy your meals even more. It can be tiresome to try to think about what meals you'll want for the week, which is why it's important to freeze meals that can last longer than a week to slowly build up your variety. Still, creating a cookbook can help you to make your meal plans easier. If you prefer freestyle cooking, then you'll also have a way to write down what ingredients you used and the rough estimate of how much.

Don't Do it Alone

If you aren't living alone, then meal prepping alone can be pointless. If you're prepping for your spouse or family, then it's easier to stick to meal prepping. You may need to make bigger batches, but it'll still be easier if your family doesn't have to cook all the time. Cleaning the kitchen will become easier too! If you have children, give them a small, easy job to do so that they can help you too, which will establish meal prepping as a relaxing and fun part of your routine.

Create a Meal Prep Box

It's best to put this box in the pantry so that you have everything you need on hand. It should be filled with your spoons, regularly used ingredients, containers and measuring cups. It's good to keep canned goods, sea salt, black pepper, herbs, spiced, olive oil, nuts and seeds. This way you have everything you need for your first meal prepping session, so you won't spend as much time looking for everything. All you'll need to add is your meat, dairy and produce. It'll make your meal prepping quicker and easier.

Don't Rush

If you have a day set aside for meal prepping, then you won't feel the need to rush. This will keep it from being a stressful experience for you. If you have other people in the kitchen talking to you, it can be even easier. Some people prefer to meal prep in the afternoon or evenings for this reason.

Breakfast Recipes

Here are some breakfast recipes to get you started! Breakfast is an important meal of the day, but so few people have the time to make anything at all. That's where meal prepping comes in handy.

1. Apple & Cinnamon Bircher Muesli

This recipe can be kept in the fridge for a few days, but it does not do well frozen. Some people even add extra nuts or seeds. You'll want to use either four small bowls or ramekins.

Serves: 4

Time: 10 Minutes

Ingredients:

- 1 ½ Cups Wholegrain Oats, Rolled
- 1 Teaspoon Ground Cinnamon
- 1 Cup Almond Milk, Unsweetened
- 2 Apples, Skin on & Grated
- 1 Cup Yogurt, Plain & Unsweetened

Directions:

1. Start by placing your yogurt, cinnamon, apple, oats, and milk in a bowl. Stir to combine it should be thick and wet. If you feel it's a little too dry, then just add a dash more milk.
2. Divide your mixture into four servings, and cover them before placing them in the fridge.
3. Serve chilled.

2. Overnight Maple Oats

This is a short term meal prep recipe since it only has one serving, but it'll still make your following day a little easier.

Serves: 1

Time: 10 Minutes

Ingredients:

- ½ Cup Rolled Oats
- ¾ Cup Almond Milk, Original
- 1 Tablespoon Chia Seeds
- 1 Tablespoon Yogurt, Plain
- ½ Teaspoon Honey, Raw
- 2 Pinches Cinnamon
- 1/8 Teaspoon Vanilla Extract, Pure

Topping:

- 1 Tablespoon Pecans, Chopped
- 1 Banana, Sliced
- 2 Teaspoon Maple syrup
- 1 Teaspoon Flaxseed, Ground

Directions:

1. In a bowl, mix everything together except your toppings and then cover it.
2. Place it in the fridge, and make sure that you leave it there for at least five hours or overnight.
3. Add your toppings right before serving.

3. Bran Muffins

You can keep these out on the counter or put them in the fridge to keep them even longer. Remember that they won't go stale nearly as quickly if you have them in an airtight container. What most people don't know is that you can freeze them too! Just allow them to cool before placing them in a freezer zip top bag. You'll either need to let them thaw the night before or microwave them for half a minute before eating them.

Serves: 12

Time: 35 Minutes

Ingredients:

- 1 Teaspoon Sea Salt, Fine
- 1 Cup Water
- 1 Cup Raisins, Pureed
- 1 ½ Cups Flour
- ¼ Cup Molasses
- ½ Cup Honey, Raw
- 1 ½ Cups Buttermilk
- 1 ½ Cups Flour
- 1 ½ Teaspoons Baking Soda
- 2 Cups Wheat Bran
- 2 Eggs, Large
- 2 ½ Tablespoons Coconut Oil, Melted

Directions:

1. Start by heating your oven to 350 degrees, and then coat a twelve cup muffin tin with your cooking spray or use paper liners.
2. Add your raisins to a saucepan with a half a cup of water, bringing it to a boil. Once it starts to boil, turn it down to simmer for ten minutes remove from heat, allowing it to cool.
3. Combine your baking soda, salt and flour in a bowl, mixing well.

4. Pulse your wheat bran and raisins in a food processor to form a crumb mixture, and then set it to the side.
5. In a large bowl, combine your bran and raisins with your honey, buttermilk and molasses. Once mixed well, add in your eggs and your remaining half a cup of water before mixing again. Add in your melted coconut oil, and stir until combined.
6. Slowly add your flour mixture in, stirring until combined.
7. Fill your muffin tins three quarters full, and then bake for twenty-five minutes. A toothpick should be able to be inserted and come out clean.

4. Tropical Smoothie Packets

You'll be creating one smoothie per packet, and you'll need to add water or milk before you can drink it, meaning you'll have to have at least five minutes for breakfast in the morning. You'll need some freezer friendly bags that are easy to seal and store.

Serves: 7

Time: 10 Minutes

Ingredients:

- 3 Cups Mixed Berries, Frozen or Fresh
- 2 Cups Kale, Chopped
- 3 Bananas, Chopped
- 2 Mangos, Fresh & Chunked

Directions:

1. Stir to combine, and then divide evenly between seven freezer bags.
2. When you're ready to make your smoothie, then just dump it into a blender and add a cup of milk or water. Coconut milk works too! Some people even like to add bit of yogurt or a handful of oats.

5. Egg & Salmon Muffins

Usually when people think of salmon, they think of sweet things, but you can have savory muffins too. You'll find these muffins are filling without being loaded in carbs. You cannot freeze these, so just store them in fridge in an airtight container.

Serves: 6

Time: 15 Minutes

Ingredients:

- 4 Eggs, Medium
- 1 Tablespoon Chives, Chopped Fine
- 1 ½ Ounces Smoked Salmon, Chopped Small
- Sea Salt & Black Pepper to Taste

Directions:

1. Start by heating your oven to 355, and then grease six muffin tins or use paper liners.
2. Place your sea salt, pepper, milk and eggs in a bowl. Beat lightly to combine, and then divide your egg mixture between your muffin tins.
3. Divide your salmon between your muffins, and then gently press it down.
4. Sprinkle the muffin mixture with your chives, and then bake for eight to ten minutes.
5. Allow it to cool for five minutes, and then store in the fridge.

6. Blueberry Bars

It's best to store these in an airtight container before placing them in the freezer. You can use these for snacks too!

Serves: 16

Time: 1 Hour 15 Minutes

Ingredients:

- 1 ½ Cups Rolled Oats
- 1/3 Cup Walnuts
- 1/3 Cup Ground Flaxseeds
- ½ Cup Pistachios, Shelled
- ½ Cup Blueberries, Dried
- ¼ Cup Sunflower Seeds
- 1/3 Cup Pumpkin Seeds
- 1/3 Cup Honey, Raw
- 1 Cup Almond Butter
- ¼ Cup Applesauce, Unsweetened

Directions:

1. Start by lining a baking pan using parchment paper. The paper should extend over the edges so it's easier to remove.
2. Combine your honey, oats, blueberries, flaxseed, pistachios, sunflower seeds, walnuts and pumpkin seeds together.
3. Stir in your almond butter and make sure it's well combined.
4. Mix all other ingredients in, and then place it in a pan. Make sure it's flat.
5. Freeze for an hour, and then peel the parchment paper off. Cut the slab into bars, and then freeze them until you're ready to eat. It's best to keep them cold.

7. Berry Chia Pots

Chia seeds are a great source of fatty acids, protein and fiber, making it the perfect energy filled breakfast ingredient. They don't do well frozen, though. So it's important to be prepared to eat them in about three days, since that's how long they'll keep in the fridge.

Serves: 5

Time: 10 Minutes

Ingredients:

- 2 Cups Mixed Berries, Fresh or Frozen
- ½ Cup Cold Water
- 1 Cup Almond Milk, Original
- 6 Tablespoons Chia Seeds
- 1 Teaspoon Vanilla Extract, Pure
- 1 Teaspoon Cinnamon
- 1 Cup Yogurt, Plain & Unsweetened

Directions:

1. Divide your berries between your pots or ramekins.
2. Get out a bowl, and then mix your almond milk, water, chia seeds, vanilla extract and cinnamon. Mix well, and then divide the chia seed mix between your pots. Spoon it on top of your berries.
3. Add in your yogurt next, and sprinkle your cinnamon on top. A few extra berries should go on top too!
4. Cover before placing in your fridge.

8. Breakfast Burritos

These will keep in the freezer for about three weeks, but some people think that they're fine for a whole month. You'll want to store them in plastic wrap and then place them in a freezer bag.

Serves: 24

Time: 20 Minutes

Ingredients:

- 24 Flour Tortillas
- 1 lb. Sausages
- 1 Bag Potato Wedges
- 12 Ounce Salsa
- 8 Eggs, Medium
- 1 Can Black Beans, Drained
- Italian Herb Seasoning

Directions:

1. Start by cooking your potato wedges using the instructions on your bag.
2. In a pan, brown your sausages, and then add in your salsa and black beans. Stir well before adding in your eggs and stirring again. Cook until your eggs are set and not runny.
3. When your wedges are done, then put them into a pan, mashing them into your mixture.
4. Season with your Italian herb seasoning, and then place three spoonfuls of the mixture into each tortilla. Roll the burrito up, and then place them on a tray. Place the tray into your freezer to cool them down before packaging.
5. To heat up your burritos, you'll need to microwave them for two minutes.

9. Green Smoothie Packets

The blueberries will make this green smoothie into a purple color, but it still is chalk full of all the nutrients that you get from your leafy greens. Just remember that you'll need to have access to a blender in the morning to make these easy meals.

Serves: 7

Time: 10 Minutes

Ingredients:

- 2 Cups Blueberries
- 4 Cups Baby Spinach, Torn
- 2 Cups Kale, Raw & Chopped
- 1 Avocado, Chunked
- 2 Green Apples, Skin On & Chunked

Directions:

1. Place your spinach, avocado, blueberries, and kale in a bowl. Stir until well combined.
2. Divide your smoothies between seven bags, sealing them and placing them in the freezer.
3. To make your smoothie, blend with water or milk.

10. Banana Pancakes

Pancakes are easy to heat up in the microwave, and with the sweet banana added in, it's up to you if you want to add syrup. The best part is that pancakes freeze well and can easily be heated up in the microwave.

Serves: 4

Time: 20 Minutes

Ingredients:

- 2 Cups Whole Wheat Flour
- 1 ½ Teaspoons Baking Soda
- 2 Teaspoon Baking Powder
- 2 Eggs, Lightly Beaten
- ½ Teaspoon Sea Salt, Fine
- 1 Tablespoon Honey, Raw
- 1 ¾ Cup Whole Milk
- 2 Tablespoons Butter, Unsalted & Melted
- Butter for Frying
- 2 Bananas, Mashed
- Pure Maple Syrup for Serving, Optional

Directions:

1. Whisk your flour, baking soda, baking powder and salt together in a large bowl.
2. Make a well in the center, and then pour in your milk, eggs, honey, and two tablespoons of melted butter. Whisk well, but make sure that you don't overmix.
3. Gently fold in your bananas after mashing them, and then heat up a sauté pan or griddle using medium-high heat swirl your butter in the pan until well coated.

4. Make your pancakes like you normally would. When they start to
   bubble, then flip it over and cook on the other side. It should take two
   to three minutes for each side.
5. Serve with maple syrup if desired.

11. Vanilla Oat Pots

This is great for active days, and will give you a generous amount of energy to get through your day. Some people prefer to add a bit of Greek yogurt to add in some extra protein too. You'll need to keep these in the fridge, since you shouldn't freeze them, but they'll keep for about four days.

Serves: 4

Time: 10 Minutes

Ingredients:

- 2 Cups Rolled Oats, Whole Grain
- 3 Teaspoons Vanilla Extract, Pure
- 3 Cups Almond Milk, Original
- 4 Prunes, Chopped Fine
- 4 Dates, Chopped Fine
- 20 Almonds, Chopped
- 12 Walnuts, Chopped

Directions:

1. Start by placing your vanilla extract, oats, almond milk, dates, prunes, almonds and walnuts in a bowl before stirring.
2. Divide your mixture between four jars, sealing and covering. Allow it to soak at least overnight.
3. Add more almond milk when serving if you feel it's too dry.

12. Smoothie Pancakes

While you can freeze these pancakes, you can also keep them in the ridge for two to three days. Just make sure to keep them in an airtight container. They add a nice twist to the usual pancake recipe, with a sweet nutty flavor due to the hemp seeds and kiwi.

Serves: 4

Time: 30 Minutes

Ingredients:

- 2 Tablespoons Maple Syrup, Optional
- 1 Tablespoon Peanut Butter
- 3 Tablespoons Hemp Seeds
- 1 Cup Baby Spinach
- ¾ Cup Vanilla Yogurt
- 2 Eggs, Medium
- 2 Kiwis, Peeled & Diced
- 1 Teaspoon Vanilla Extract, Pure
- 1 Teaspoon Baking Powder
- 1 Teaspoon Cinnamon
- 1 Cup Whole Wheat Flour

Directions:

1. Start by processing your spinach, vanilla extract, yogurt, hemp seeds, peanut butter, eggs, kiwis, and maple syrup together. Blend well.
2. Add in your baking powder, flour and cinnamon, blending until mixed well.
3. Cook your pancakes in a griddle, and serve topped with yogurt or syrup.
4. You can freeze them ahead of time, and microwave them for one to two minutes to serve.

13. Breakfast Peppers

When most people think of stuffed bell peppers, they think of dinner. Of course, this recipe is great for breakfast, and it's easy to freeze. Just make sure that you freeze each pepper in an individual container so that they don't tear when you're removing them to heat up.

Serves: 3

Time: 35 Minutes

Ingredients:

- 9 Eggs, Large
- 4 Bell Peppers, Whatever Color
- ½ Cup Breakfast Potatoes, Cooked
- ½ Cup Quinoa, Cooked
- ½ Cup Black Beans
- 1/3 Cup Cheese, Shredded + Cheese for Topping
- ½ Cup Spinach, Chopped
- 1 Teaspoon Sea Salt, Fine
- ¼ Teaspoon Black Pepper

Directions:

1. Start by heating your oven to 400, and then cut your peppers in half. Remove the seeds, and then place them on a baking sheet. Bake for five minutes.
2. Crack your eggs into a bowl, and beat them lightly.
3. Add in all of your ingredients, mixing until combined well.
4. Remove your peppers from the oven, placing the mixture inside of each one.
5. Sprinkle with cheese and black pepper before placing it back in the oven.

6. Bake for twenty minutes, and then serve immediately or keep in an airtight container in the fridge. You can freeze them, but it may change the texture of your eggs.

14. Chicken Breakfast Casseroles

You'll want to cook your casserole, let it cool down, and then cut it into the proper portions before freezing it. You can also decide to keep it in the fridge, but unless you're feeding more than one person placing it in the freezer is best.

Serves: 4

Time: 40 Minutes

Ingredients:

- 2 Rashers Bacon, Diced
- 2 Cloves Garlic, Minced
- 1 lb. Chicken Breast, Diced
- ½ Cup Onion, Diced
- 1 Red Pepper, Diced
- 2 Cups Spinach
- 1 Large Sweet Potato, Peeled & Spiralized
- ½ Cup Water
- 1 Teaspoon Paprika
- ½ Teaspoon Cayenne Pepper
- 1 Teaspoon All Purpose Seasoning
- 6 Eggs, Medium

Directions:

1. Start by sautéing your onion, peppers, bacon, garlic, sweet potato and chicken together in a pan until your chicken is cooked all the way through. Add in your water, spinach and seasoning, cooking or another three minutes.
2. Transfer the mixture to a greased nine by nine pan, and then whisk your eggs together in a bowl. Pour your eggs over the mixture.
3. Set your oven to 375 degrees, and then bake for twenty minutes while covered with foil.

4. Take the cover of, and then cook for another ten minutes.

5. Allow it to cool before slicing, and then package as desired.

Snack Recipes

While you can use some of the breakfast recipes for snacks as well, you'll find you still need to prep some snack recipes to keep you from leaning towards unhealthy foods.

15. Cornmeal & Apple Muffins

Remember that you can freeze your muffins, so there's no reason to try to eat all twelve in just a few days. However, remember that they'll need time to thaw if you don't have access to a microwave.

Serves: 12

Time: 35 Minutes

Ingredients:

- ¾ Cup Applesauce
- ¼ Cup Coconut Oil, Melted
- ½ Cup Apple Cider
- ¼ Cup Maple Syrup
- 2 Eggs
- 1 ½ Cups Oat Flour
- ½ Cup Cornmeal, Ground
- ½ Teaspoon Sea Salt, Fine
- ½ Teaspoon Baking Soda
- ½ Teaspoon Cinnamon
- 1 Cup Apple, Peeled & Chopped
- ¼ Cup Apple Chips, Dried & Chopped

Directions:

1. Start by heating your oven to 350, and then take out a bowl.
2. Mix your coconut oil, apple cider, eggs, applesauce, and maple syrup together. Make sure it's whisked well.

3. Add in your apple chips, oat flour, sea salt, baking soda, cornmeal and cinnamon, stirring well.
4. Grease a muffin pan, and then spoon two tablespoons of batter into each one.
5. Bake for twenty-five minutes. A toothpick should come out clean when inserted into the middle.
6. Allow to cool before packaging.

16. Chai & Maple Chickpeas

These roasted chickpeas are easy to take on the go, and you can freeze them without changing their flavor or texture.

Serves: 6

Time: 50 Minutes

Ingredients:

- 2 Cups Chickpeas, Drained, Rinsed & Dried
- 1 Tablespoon Olive Oil
- 1 Tablespoon Maple Syrup, Pure
- ½ Teaspoon Ginger, Ground
- ½ Teaspoon Cinnamon
- ¼ Teaspoon Cardamom
- ¼ Teaspoon Cloves
- ¼ Teaspoon Sea Salt, Fine
- ¼ Teaspoon Black Pepper

Directions:

1. Start by heating your oven to 400 degrees.
2. In a bowl, toss your chickpeas with your maple syrup, cinnamon, oil, ginger, cloves, cardamom, salt and pepper.
3. Spread them on a baking sheet, making sure it's a single layer. Bake your chickpeas for thirty-five to thirty-eight minutes. You'll need to shake your baking sheet every ten minutes to make sure that they cook evenly.
4. Allow to cool before packaging.

17. Cheese & Leek Muffins

This is another example of a savory muffin that's a healthy snacking option, which can be kept at room temperature, in the fridge or frozen, depending on how quickly you think you'll go through them. They can technically be used as a side dish for dinner too. Some people even use them for breakfast.

Serves: 9

Time: 35 Minutes

Ingredients:

- 1 Cup Flour, Plain
- 1 Teaspoon Baking Powder
- ¼ Teaspoon Bicarbonate Soda
- ¼ Cup Milk
- ½ Teaspoon Allspice
- 1 Egg, Beaten
- ½ Cup Vegetable Oil
- 1 Leek, Diced
- 3 Ounces Cheddar, Grated

Directions:

1. Start by heating your oven to 360, and then combine all of your dry ingredients into a bowl.
2. Gently stir in your oil, egg and milk into your dry ingredients.
3. Add in your diced leek and cheddar, stirring well.
4. Grease your muffin tray before spooning the mixture into it.
5. Bake for twenty to twenty-five minutes.
6. Allow it to cool before packaging.

18. Apple Pie Balls

These are another type of energy balls which taste like apple pie, which is a healthy alternative to a slice of apple pie in the middle of the day.

Serves: 15

Time: 10 Minutes

Ingredients:

- 1 Cup Dates, Pitted
- 1 Cup Cashews
- 1 Cup Apple Rings, Unsweetened, Dried & Chopped
- ½ Cup Rolled Oats
- 1 Teaspoon Cinnamon
- ¼ Teaspoon Sea Salt, Fine
- ¼ Teaspoon Nutmeg

Directions:

1. Place your cashews, dates, and apple rings in a food processor. Allow it to form into a sticky substance, and then add in your spices, salt, and oats. Pulse until mixed well.
2. Portion into balls, and roll them in the palm of your hand
3. These energy balls will store safely in your fridge or two weeks, or you can keep them even longer in the freezer.

19. Fruit & Oat Cookies

These healthy cookies are meant to help with sweet carvings, and they're a healthy alternative to traditional cookies. Some people even use them to go with their breakfast if they're still hungry, but you can freeze them!

Serves: 24

Time: 15 Minutes

Ingredients:

- ½ Cup Flour, Whole meal
- 1 Teaspoon Mixed Spices
- ½ Teaspoon Bicarbonate Soda
- 2 Cps Porridge Oats
- 2 Tablespoons Mixed Seeds
- ½ Cup Dried Fruit, Chopped
- ½ Cup Butter, Unsalted
- ½ Cup Brown Sugar
- 1 Egg, Medium

Directions:

1. Start by heating your oven to 350.
2. In a bowl combine your mixed spices, flour, oats, bicarbonate soda, seeds and dried fruit. Mix well.
3. Cream your butter in a different bowl, and then stir in your sugar. Continue to stir until light and fluffy, and then add in your egg. Beat to combine.
4. Add in your oat mixture, and then wet your hands. Roll the sticky mixture into balls, and then place them on a tray.
5. Bake for eight to ten minutes, cooking until lightly browned
6. You can store them in the fridge or at room temperature in an airtight container for five days.

20. Chocolate Energy Balls

If you're looking for a snack to give you a natural pick-me-up, then this is a snack for you! They're easy to make, and it only takes a minute to pop one out of the fridge. It's best not to freeze them, or you'll change the texture.

Serves: 10

Time: 10 Minutes

Ingredients:

- ½ Cup Pitted Dates, Soft
- ½ Cup Almonds, Raw
- 1 Tablespoon Matcha Green Tea Powder
- Matcha Green Tea Powder for Dusting
- ¼ Cup Cocoa powder, Unsweetened
- 1 Tablespoon Almond Milk, Unsweetened

Directions:

1. Add your almonds and dates into a food processor, and process until they come together. Add in your matcha powder, cocoa powder and almond milk, blending until you have a thick, smooth consistency. It should have a similar consistency to ganache.

2. Portion the mixture into ten servings, and roll them into balls with the palm of your hand. Dust your balls with matcha powder, and then store in your refrigerator for up to two weeks.

21. Vanilla & Lemon Balls

These are another energy ball that keeps for a long time in the fridge. You can keep them in the fridge for two weeks or freeze them to keep them even later.

Serves: 20

Time: 10 Minutes

Ingredients:

- 1 Cup Almonds, Raw
- ½ Cup Vanilla Protein Powder
- 1 Cup Dates, Pitted
- 2 Teaspoon Maca Powder
- ½ Teaspoon Sea Salt, Fine
- 1 Lemon, Zested
- ½ Lemon, Juiced

Directions:

1. Place your almonds in a food processor, and then process until it turns crumbly.
2. Add your protein powder, maca powder and dates, processing until combined well.
3. Add your lemon juice, lemon zest, and sea salt. Process until it turns into a sticky, thick mixture.
4. Roll into balls in your hand, and then store properly.

22. Sweet Potato Cookies

These healthy cookies are filled with protein, and they can be kept in the fridge for four days or frozen. Just make sure that you let them thaw overnight before eating if you freeze them.

Serves: 8

Time: 15 Minutes

Ingredients:

- 1 Cup Sweet Potato, Cooked & Mashed
- ½ Cup Nut Butter
- 1 Teaspoon Vanilla Extract, Pure
- 2 Eggs, Medium
- 1 Teaspoon Cinnamon
- 2 Tablespoons Maple Syrup
- 2 Tablespoons Chia Seeds
- ½ Cup Pepitas
- ¼ Cup Craisins
- ¼ Cup Oat Flour
- 1 Teaspoon Baking Soda

Directions:

1. Combine your sweet potato, eggs and nut butter in a bowl before mixing well.
2. Add in your baking soda, vanilla extract, oat flour, maple syrup, cinnamon, chia seeds, Craisins and Pepitas. Stir well.
3. Roll the mixture into balls, and flatten them slightly with your palm before placing them on a baking sheet that's been lined with parchment paper.
4. Bake at 375 for about ten minutes. They should become lightly browned.
5. Allow to cool before packaging properly.

23. Apricot Energy Bars

These energy bars are easy to make, and they're versatile too. You can use other dried fruit for different flavors, such as strawberries, blueberries or even cranberries. They store well either in the freezer or in your fridge.

Serves: 12

Time: 15 Minutes

Ingredients:

- 1 Cup Pitted Dates, Whole
- 1 Cup Apricots, Dried
- 1 Cup Almonds, Chopped
- 2 Scoops Protein Powder, Vanilla

Directions:

1. Place your apricots, almonds, and dates in a food processor, pulsing for one to two minutes. You'll need to scrape the sides of your bowl every once in a while to keep it from sticking.
2. Add your protein powder in, and then process for another two to three minutes. The mixture should become crumbly and sticky.
3. Use plastic wrap to line a shallow pan, and then add in your mixture. Press until flat, and then cover, refrigerating for an hour.
4. Take them on of the fridge and cut the slab into twelve bars.
5. Store up to one week in the fridge, or package them for freezing.

24. Easy Hummus

This is an everyday hummus recipe which can be served with pretzels or crackers. You can even serve it with fresh vegetables. You'll need to give it time to thaw if you freeze it!

Serves: 4

Time: 10 Minutes

Ingredients:

- 32 Ounces Garbanzo Beans, Reduced Sodium, Rinsed & Drained Reserve ¼ Cup Liquid
- 1 Tablespoon Olive Oil
- ¼ Cup Lemon Juice
- 2 Cloves Garlic, Minced
- ¼ Teaspoon Black Pepper
- ¼ Teaspoon Paprika
- 3 Tablespoons Tahini
- 2 Tablespoons Flat Leaf Parsley, Chopped

Directions:

1. Start by adding your beans into a processor, pureeing until smooth.
2. Add in your lemon juice, garlic, olive oil, paprika, parsley, pepper and tahini, blending until smooth.
3. Pour in your reserved liquid a tablespoon at a time until you have a thick spread.
4. Either freeze in individual servings or keep in the fridge for three to four days.

Side Dish Recipes

Everyone needs side dishes, but you can make these in advance too! Most meal prepping meals will be a one pot dish, but this isn't always the case. That's where these recipes come in handy.

25. Coleslaw

Most people won't use this as a snack, but it makes a great side dish! Just make sure that you package it separately from the rest of your food.

Serves: 4

Time: 1 Hour 10 Minutes

Ingredients:

- 1 Cabbage Head, Shredded
- 2 Cups Sugar
- 1 Teaspoon Sea Salt, Fine
- 1 Cup Vinegar
- 1 Green Pepper, Seeded & Chopped
- 1 Carrot, Shredded
- 1 Teaspoon Dry Mustard
- 1 Teaspoon Celery Seeds

Directions:

1. Combine your green pepper, cabbage, salt and carrot together in a bowl. Let it sit for an hour.
2. Add all remaining ingredients into a saucepan before bringing it to a boil. Reduce it to a simmer, allowing it to cook for two minutes.
3. Drain your vegetables, and then add it to your vinegar mixture, mixing well.
4. Allow it to cool before freezing. Serve chilled, but make sure that it's completely thawed!

26. Garlic Mash

Mashed potatoes heat up great in the microwave, making them the perfect side dish to meal prep!

Serves: 6

Time: 20 Minutes

Ingredients:

- 2 Cups Whole Milk
- ½ Tablespoon Sea Salt, Fine
- 6 Cloves Garlic, Minced
- 3 ½ lbs. Russet Potatoes
- 6 Ounces Shaved Parmesan

Directions:

1. Start by peeling and dicing your potatoes. It's best if they're all the same size.
2. Put your potatoes in a saucepan, covering it with water and adding your salt.
3. Bring the saucepan to a boil, cooking until your potatoes break down easily when poked with a fork.
4. Drain your potatoes off, setting them to the side. You'll want to give them some time to steam dry too.
5. Heat your garlic and milk in a different saucepan, cooking until it simmers. Set it to the side.
6. Add you garlic and milk mixture to your potatoes, and then add in the cheese. Make sure to stir to combine, and mash if necessary.
7. Freeze after it cools.

27. Roasted Carrots

Carrots freeze and heat up well, making them a great meal prepping food.

Serves: 4

Time: 30 Minutes

Ingredients:

- 1 Tablespoon Olive Oil
- ½ Teaspoon Paprika
- 8 Carrots
- Sea Salt & Black Pepper to Taste

Directions:

1. Start by heating your oven to 425.
2. Cut your carrots into one inch slices, and then take out a bowl.
3. Whisk your olive oil, paprika, sea salt and black pepper together.
4. Pour this mixture over your carrots, tossing to coat
5. Bake for twenty minutes, and stir halfway through. Your carrots should be tender but crisp.
6. Allow your carrots to cool before portioning them out and freezing them.

28. Celeriac Mash

If you're looking for an alternative to mashed potatoes that freezes well, try this celeriac mash which has a slight natural sweetness due to the carrots and apple.

Serves: 6

Time: 30 Minutes

Ingredients:

- 1 ½ lbs. Celeriac, Chopped
- 4 Apples, Peeled & Cubed
- 2 lbs. Carrots, Peeled & Sliced
- 4 Tablespoons Crème Fraiche
- 1 Tablespoon Butter, Melted
- 4 Tablespoon Parsley, Fresh & Chopped

Directions:

1. Start by bringing a pot of water to a boil, adding in your apples, carrots and celeriac. Simmer until tender, which should take about twenty minutes.
2. Drain the water off, and then put your vegetables and apple back in the pot. Add your crème fraiche, parsley and butter before mashing all of your ingredients together.
3. Freeze once cool.

29. Lemon Green Beans

Green beans are another vegetable that heat up well after being frozen, making them a great meal prepping side dish to pair with your choice of protein.

Serves: 4

Time: 15 Minutes

Ingredients:

- 1 lb. Green Beans, Stems Removed
- 2 Tablespoons Olive Oil
- ½ Teaspoon Lemon Zest
- 1 Clove Garlic, Minced
- Sea Salt & Black Pepper
- Fresh Lemon Juice to Taste

Directions:

1. Start by bringing a pot of water to boil, and then add in your green beans.
2. In a bowl, mix your garlic and olive oil together. Add in your lemon zest and a few squeezes of a lemon wedge. Season with salt and pepper, mixing well.
3. Continue to boil your green beans until they're tender, and then drain them.
4. Rinse your green beans under cold water, and allow them to steam dry for two to three minutes before transferring them to a bowl.
5. Toss your green beans with your lemon juice mixture, and allow them to cool before portioning them out to freeze.

30. Easy Asparagus

When people think of a quick, easy vegetable that freezes well, most people skip over asparagus even though they're a great choice.

Serves: 4

Time: 15 Minutes

Ingredients:

- 1 lb. Asparagus
- 2 Teaspoons Olive Oil
- ½ Teaspoon Smoked Paprika
- Sea Salt & Black Pepper to Taste

Directions:

1. Start by heating your oven to 400, and then trim the tough ends off of your asparagus.
2. Place your asparagus on a baking sheet, and then toss them in your olive oil. Sprinkle your seasonings over them, making sure your asparagus is in a single layer.
3. Roast your asparagus until tender, which should take ten to fifteen minutes depending on thickness.
4. Allow your asparagus to cool before freezing. Cutting your roasted asparagus in half will make it easier to eat on the go!

Lunch Recipes

Lunch can be one of the hardest meals to carve out time for, which is why meal prepping is needed. Most of these recipes can be kept in the fridge for a few days, but you can also freeze a large majority of them. Make the recipes that fit into your busy schedule.

31. Greens & Quinoa Salad

You'll want airtight containers to store this in the fridge, but quinoa isn't just a specialty ingredient. It makes a great salad that's full of the fiber and protein you need to get through the day.

Serves: 4

Time: 25 Minutes

Ingredients:

- 1 Cup Quinoa, Dry
- 12 Ounces Chicken Stock
- 3 Cups Lettuce, Shredded
- 2 Cups Baby Spinach Leaves
- 3 Ounces Feta, Small Chunks
- 2 Green Bell Peppers, Cored, Seeded & Sliced
- Sea Salt & Black Pepper to Taste

Directions:

1. Make sure to rinse your quinoa before starting, and then bring the chicken broth to a boil. Once it starts to boil add in your quinoa, stirring to combine.
2. Reduce it to a simmer, and cover it. Cook for about twelve to fifteen minutes. Your liquid should have disappeared, leaving you a soft quinoa.
3. Divide the quinoa between four different airtight containers, and then divide the rest of your ingredients.

4. Sprinkle with salt and pepper and drizzle with olive oil if desired.

5. Cover, placing it in the fridge until you're ready to use it.

32. Potato & Sausage Pockets

You can freeze these just like you would Hot Pockets, and they're a much healthier alternative!

Serves: 6

Time: 1 Hour

Ingredients:

- ½ lb. Mushrooms, Diced
- ½ lb. Potatoes, Sliced Thin
- 6 Ounces Chicken Sausage, Cooked & Sliced
- Sea Salt & Black Pepper to Taste
- 10 Ounces Spinach, Fresh & Chopped
- 2 Tablespoons Olive Oil
- 1 Cup Cheddar Cheese, Grated
- 1 lb. Pizza Dough, Whole Wheat & Room Temperature
- Flour for Your Surface

Directions:

1. Start by heating your oven to 400
2. Line a baking tray with parchment paper, and then toss on your sausage, potatoes, mushrooms onto it. Sprinkle with oil and season with salt and pepper.
3. Place your tray in the oven, roasting for twenty-five minutes. Your potatoes should become tender, allowing it to cool before transferring it to a bowl.
4. Mix in your spinach and cheese.
5. Lightly flour a surface, and then separate your dough into six pieces. Roll each piece into a six inch round.
6. Spoon your mixture into the center of each, and then fold the dough over after dampening the edge with water. Press closed.

7. Cut slits into the tops of each pocket, baking for about twenty
   minutes. They should become a golden brown.
8. To heat up, allow them to cook in the microwave for about two
   minutes.

33. Meatball Bowl

Serves: 4

Time: 1 Hour 10 Minutes

Ingredients:

- 2 Cups Brown Rice
- 2 Tablespoons Basil, Chopped Fine
- 2 Tablespoon Cilantro, Chopped Fine
- 2 Tablespoons Mint, Chopped Fine
- 2 Tablespoons Green Onions, Fresh & Diced
- ¼ Cup Peanuts, Crushed
- Sriracha to Taste

Pickled Carrots:

- 1/3 Cup Rice Vinegar
- 1 Tablespoon Sesame Oil
- 1 Teaspoon Sea Salt, Fine
- ¼ Cup Coconut Palm Sugar
- 6 Carrots, Cut into Thin Ribbons

Meatballs:

- 4 Cloves Garlic, Minced
- 1 Tablespoon Chili Paste
- 1 Tablespoon Fish Sauce
- 2 Tablespoons Lemongrass Paste
- 1 lb. Ground Pork
- 1 Tablespoon Coconut Palm Sugar
- 1 Teaspoon Sea Salt, Fine
- 2 Teaspoons Cornstarch

Directions:

1. Start by preparing your pickled carrots. Whisk your palm sugar, sesame oil, salt and vinegar together. Soak your carrots in this mixture for about an hour.
2. Prepare your meatballs next by mixing all of the ingredients together, and then roll the mixture into small balls with your hands.
3. Heat a bit of your olive oil in a skillet using medium-high heat, and then fry your meatballs until golden brown. They should be cooked all the way through.
4. Layer your carrots and meatballs over your rice, topping with your chopped herbs and peanuts.
5. Keep your sriracha separate until you go to serve it. Remember that you can keep it in the fridge or freezer depending on your preference.

34. Roasted Vegetable Salad

If you're looking for a vegetable dish that's served hot, then this is dish for you! It will heat up just fine, so feel free to keep it in the fridge or freezer.

Serves: 4

Time: 30 Minutes

Ingredients:

- 2 Cups Butternut Squash, Skin On
- 2 Cups Sweet Potato, Cubed
- 2 Portobello Mushrooms, Large & Sliced Thick
- 2 Carrots, Chunked
- 2 Zucchinis, Large & Chunked
- 2 Tablespoons Sunflower Seeds
- 2 Tablespoons Pumpkin Seeds
- 1 Head Broccoli, Chopped into Florets
- 3 Tablespoons Olive Oil
- Sea Salt & Black Pepper to Taste

Directions:

1. Start by heating your oven to 356 degrees, and then line a tray with baking paper.
2. Place all ingredients onto the tray, sprinkling it with your salt and pepper.
3. Combine your ingredients together, making sure it's well coated in oil.
4. Bake for thirty minutes in the oven. Your vegetables should tender, and the seeds should be toasted.
5. Allow it to cool before dividing it between your containers.

35. Fajita Bowl

You can freeze this bowl, but it's best to use airtight containers such as glass, since it can take a while to heat up. You'll want to heat it up for two minutes, stir and then heat it up for another one to two minutes in the microwave. Alternatively, you can keep it in the fridge since it only makes four servings. Either way, remember to keep your vinaigrette separately.

Serves: 4

Time: 30 Minutes

Ingredients:

- 1 Tablespoon Olive Oil
- ¾ Cup Basmati Rice, Uncooked
- 2 Bell Peppers, Sliced into Strips
- Sea Salt & Black Pepper to Taste
- 2 Chicken Breasts
- 2 Tablespoons Red Onion, Diced
- 1 Cup Corn Kernels

Vinaigrette:

- 1 Teaspoon Chili Powder
- 1 Tablespoon Sugar
- ½ Teaspoon Paprika
- 1 Tablespoon Lime Juice
- ½ Teaspoon Ground Cumin
- ¼ Teaspoon Sea Salt, Fine
- 3 Tablespoons Olive Oil
- 3 Tablespoons White Wine Vinegar

Directions:

1. Start by heating your oven to 425, and then place your chicken in a baking dish. Sprinkle your salt and pepper over your chicken before drizzling them with olive oil. Flip them over and repeat.

2. Bake your chicken for twenty minutes, but make sure you turn them over halfway through to make sure your meat is cooked all the way through.

3. Allow your chicken to cool for ten minutes, and then slice it.

4. Cook your rice according to the instructions on the package, allowing it to cool.

5. Whisk all of your vinaigrette ingredients in a bowl.

6. Spoon your rice into bowls, topping with bell pepper. Fill another bowl red onion and corn, tossing everything to mix it.

7. Portion your rice and vegetables together among your bowls and then top with chicken.

8. Store until you're ready to serve.

36. Burrito Bowl

This pork burrito bowl is best if kept in the fridge due to the lettuce, but you can always skip that part and just top with lettuce before serving if you prefer to keep it in the freezer.

Serves: 4

Time: 2 Hours 15 Minutes

Ingredients:

- 1 Can Yellow Sweet Corn
- 1 Can Black Beans, Rinsed & Drained
- 4 Cups Romaine Lettuce, Chopped
- 2 Cups Brown Rice, Cooked
- ¼ Cup Cilantro, Chopped Fine
- 1/3 Cup Red Onion, Chopped Fine
- 1/3 Cup Cojita Cheese
- ½ Teaspoon Paprika
- 2 Limes
- Sea Salt & Black Pepper to Taste

Carnitas:

- 1 lb. Pork Loin
- 1 Tablespoon Orange Juice
- 1 Tablespoon Garlic, Minced
- 1/3 Cup Lime Juice
- 3 Teaspoons Cumin
- 2 Teaspoons Smoked Paprika
- ¼ Cup Green Chilies
- Sea Salt & Black Pepper to Taste

Directions:

1. Start by placing your garlic and pork loin into a crock pot, cooking for two to four hours on high.

2. Remove your pork loin, allowing it to cool enough to shred it. Place the pork in a bowl, and mix the rest of your carnitas ingredients. Make sure that it's all mixed well.

3. In a bowl combine your corn, cojita cheese, juice from half of a lime, red onion and paprika together.

4. In a different bowl toss your rice with the juice from half a lime, and then add in your cilantro. Mix again.

5. Assemble your bowls by lining the bottom with your lettuce, and then top with your rice mixture. Put your carnitas mixture on top, and then add in your corn and black beans. Serve with a lime wedge.

6. Store in airtight containers either in the fridge or freezer.

37. Tuna Bowl

This is a heart healthy lunch that can be prepared in advance, and it's affordable too!

Serves: 4

Time: 25 Minutes

Ingredients:

- 2 Cups Brown Rice, Dry
- 4 small Cans Tuna, Unflavored
- 1 Carrot, Chopped & Peeled
- 1 Red Bell Pepper, Cored, Seeded & Chopped
- 1 Cup Cucumber, Chopped
- 1 Tablespoon Balsamic Vinegar

Directions:

1. Put your brown rice in a pot, adding three and a half cups of water and just a pinch of salt. Allow it to come to a boil, and then reduce it to a simmer. Cover and cook until your rice is soft and no water is rest.
2. Divide your rice between your containers, and then top with your tuna. Divide your cucumber, carrot and bell pepper between your bowls.
3. If you're freezing it, do not add your balsamic vinegar until after you heat it up again.

38. Salmon with Greens

This is another recipe that will keep in the fridge for three to five days, but it shouldn't be frozen or you'll get wilted greens.

Serves: 4

Time: 30 Minutes

Ingredients:

- 4 Small Salmon Fillets
- Olive Oil to Taste
- 1 Head Broccoli, Chopped into Florets
- Sea Salt & Black Pepper to Taste
- 2 Zucchinis, Chopped
- 1 Teaspoon Sesame Oil

Directions:

1. Start by eating your oven to 355, and then line a sheet with parchment paper.
2. Put your salmon filets down, and sprinkle with salt and pepper. Drizzle your olive oil over your salmon fillets.
3. Bake your salmon in the oven for about twelve minutes.
4. Put a pot of water over high heat, letting it boil. Put a steamer basket in your pot, and then put your greens inside. Put your lid on the basket.
5. Steam your vegetables until cooked all the way through. This should take three to five minutes.
6. Take them out, and then sprinkle your greens with salt, pepper and sesame oil.
7. Put your salmon fillets into your containers. Divide your vegetables between the containers too.
8. Allow it to cool before securing the lid, and serve either hot or cold.

39. Hawaiian Chicken Bowls

This noodle and chicken bowl is sweet and healthy, making it the perfect but filling bowl to take with you on the go. Remember that you shouldn't freeze pasta!

Serves: 4

Time: 2 Hours

Ingredients:

- 4 Cups Rice Noodles, Cooked
- 1 Cup Pineapple, Fresh & Cubed
- ½ Cup Pineapple Juice
- 4 Small Chicken Breasts, Skinless & Boneless
- 2 Tablespoons Ketchup
- 1 Teaspoon Garlic, Minced
- ½ Teaspoon Ginger, Fresh & Grated
- 2 Tablespoons Tamari, Low Sodium
- 1 Tablespoon Honey, Raw
- Coconut Chips to Taste
- Green Onion, Diced for Garnish
- Sea Salt to Taste

Pineapple Stir Fry:

- 1 Tablespoon Coconut Oil
- 1 Cup Purple Onion, Diced
- 2 Sweet Peppers, Large & Diced
- 2 Cups Kale, Chopped & Packed
- 1 Tablespoon Pineapple Juice
- 1 Tablespoon Chili Sauce
- 1 Tablespoon Tamari, Low Sodium
- ½ Tablespoon Honey, Raw
- 1 Tablespoon Garlic, Minced

Directions:

1. Get out a bowl and whisk your ketchup, ginger, garlic, pineapple juice, honey, salt and tamari together. Put your chicken breasts into a crock pot, and pour the sauce over it.
2. Cook your chicken for one and a half to two hours on high, and then shred it.
3. Heat a tablespoon of your coconut oil in a skillet, adding in your pepper and onions. Sauté until your onions turn translucent, and then add in your kale. Sauté or a few more minutes until wilted.
4. Mix the rest of your ingredients in a bowl, pouring it over your stir fry. Cook for a few minutes. Your sauce should reduce, and then you're ready to assemble your bowls.
5. Add your noodles to the bottom, and top with your pineapple. Add your shredded chicken next.
6. Place your pineapple stir fry on top, and then sprinkle in your green onions and coconut chips.

40. Smoked Salmon Wraps

It's best to use wholegrain wraps to make this even healthier! You can actually freeze these, and it shouldn't cause an issue. Just heat up in the microwave for thirty seconds to forty-five seconds to get the chill off.

Serves: 4

Time: 20 Minutes

Ingredients:

- 4 Wraps, Wholegrain
- 2 Avocados, Sliced Fresh
- 2 Cups Lettuce, Sliced
- 3 Ounces Smoked Salmon
- Olive Oil to Taste
- 1 Tablespoon Balsamic Vinegar
- 1 Tablespoon Olive Oil

Directions:

1. Mix your balsamic vinegar and olive oil together, and then set it to the side.
2. Put your wraps on a board, and then pile your lettuce on each one.
3. Add ½ an avocado top after slicing it, and drizzle with your olive oil and vinegar. Add your smoked salmon on top, and then wrap your wraps up.
4. Store them in the fridge or freezer.

41. Quinoa & Coconut Bowls

These quinoa bowls pack a lot of flavor, and quinoa is easy to heat up. If you're worried about your quinoa getting too mushy, then package your thinned peanut butter on the side. Only place it on after your meal is thawed or heated up as desired.

Serves: 4

Time: 45 Minutes

Ingredients:

- 1 Can Coconut Milk
- ½ Cup Water
- 2 Cups Quinoa
- 1 Sweet Potato, Large & Diced
- 2 Cups Carrot, Diced
- 2 Tablespoons Olive Oil
- 1 Tablespoon Garlic, Minced
- ¼ Cup Peanut Butter
- 2 Tablespoons Peanuts, Crushed
- Sea Salt & Black Pepper to Taste
- 2 Tablespoons Cilantro, Chopped Fine

Cabbage Slaw:

- 1 Cup Purple Cabbage, Chopped Fine
- 1 Cup Edamame
- 1 Red Pepper, Small & Diced
- 1 Tablespoon Tamari, Low Sodium
- 2 Tablespoon Olive Oil
- ¼ Teaspoon Garlic Powder
- 1 Lime, Juiced
- 1 Tablespoon Maple Syrup
- ¼ Teaspoon Orange Peel, Dried

- ¼ Teaspoon Ginger Powder

Directions:

1. In a medium pot bring your coconut milk, quinoa and water to a boil. Once it starts to boil reduce it to low, and then cover. Cook for about ten minutes. All of your liquid should be absorbed, and then season with sea salt and black pepper. Fluff with a fork, and set your quinoa to the side.
2. Place your vegetables on a baking sheet, drizzling your olive oil over them. Mix in your garlic before seasoning with your salt and pepper. Make sure it's coated well.
3. Roast at 400 for twenty-five to thirty minutes. Your vegetables should become tender
4. In a bowl, mix your cabbage, red pepper and edamame. Mix all remaining cabbage slaw ingredients together, tossing until everything is well coated.
5. To assemble your bowls add your quinoa on the bottom. Top with your roasted vegetables and slaw.
6. Sprinkle your cilantro and peanuts on top, and then thin your peanut butter out with olive oil. Drizzle this on top of your bowls.
7. Make sure everything is cool before packaging for your fridge or freezer.

42. Stuffed Sweet Potatoes

Sweet potatoes are easy to keep in the fridge, but it is best you do not freeze these. Keep this recipe in the fridge until you're ready to eat it!

Serves: 4

Time: 20 Minutes

Ingredients:

- 4 Sweet Potatoes, Pricked with a Fork
- Handful Parsley, Chopped Fine
- 1 Scallion, Chopped Fine
- 1 Cup Cottage Cheese
- 1 Cup Baby Spinach Leaves
- Sea Salt & Black Pepper to Taste

Directions:

1. Microwave your sweet potatoes on high for a full minute.
2. Cut them in half, removing the flesh. Reserve the flesh in a bowl, and then add your spinach, parsley, spinach, scallions, salt and pepper to the bowl. Stir to combine.
3. Fill your sweet potatoes skins back up with the mixture.
4. Package two halves in each of your four containers before placing them in the fridge.

Dinner Recipes

Most of the time if you have a busy schedule, it can be just as hard to cook dinner. After all, you'll want a little me time, which can't happen if you're busy cooking on your time off. Try these dinner recipes instead!

43. Pumpkin & Coconut Soup

This is a simple freezer soup recipe, and it's easy to store! It heats up well, and it's satisfying during any time of the year. The best part is that it's low in calories too!

Serves: 6

Time: 45 Minutes

Ingredients:

- 1 Onion, Chopped Fine
- 6 Cups Pumpkin, Skinned & Cubed
- 2 Carrots, Chunked
- 1 Cup Coconut Milk
- 3 Cups Chicken Stock
- Sea Salt & Black Pepper to Taste

Directions:

1. Put your onion, carrots, pumpkin, sea salt, pepper and stock into a pot, bringing it all to a boil. Reduce the temperature to let it simmer, and then cover the pot. Cook while covered or twenty-five minutes. Your vegetables should become tender.
2. Use an immersion blender, and then blend until smooth.
3. Stir in your coconut milk, and then add salt and pepper as desired.
4. Allow your soup to cool, and then pour into six containers.
5. Freeze your containers until they're needed.

44. Bourguignon

This beef dish is a great dinner, and it's hearty to keep you full. It's great to freeze and pop it out later. It's best to pop it in the oven for twenty to thirty minutes to heat it back up.

Serves: 6

Time: 2 Hours 20 Minutes

Ingredients:

- 1 lb. Chuck Roast, Boneless & Cubed
- 2 Cups Beef Stock
- 4 Ounces Bacon
- ¼ Teaspoon Thyme, Dried
- ¼ Teaspoon Black Pepper
- 1 Bay Leaf
- 1 ½ Cups Dry Red Wine
- ¼ Cup Flour, Plain
- 2 Cups White Mushrooms, Sliced
- 1 Brown Onion, Sliced

Directions:

1. Start by heating your oven to 340, and then cut your bacon into half inch strips. Cook your bacon until crisp.
2. Put your bacon in a baking dish, making sure to reserve the fat separately.
3. Brown your roast, making sure you brown it on all sides, using your bacon grease. Place your chuck on the bacon.
4. Add in your flour to the remaining fat, and then stir. Use medium heat, cooking until your flour has browned. It should dissolve completely.
5. Add in your stock and wine slowly, stirring to make sure that it doesn't have any lumps. Add the thyme, pepper and bay leaf, allowing it to simmer for five minutes. It should thicken slightly.

6. Pour your mixture over your roast, and then cover it. Bake for one and a half hours. Your chuck should become tender.

7. Remove the dish, stirring in your mushrooms and onions.

8. Bake for another hour, and then serve with a side of either potatoes or rice.

9. Allow it to cool before you freeze them.

45. Easy Shepherd's Pie

If you like traditional shepherd's pie, then this is the recipe for you. It's easy to make and tastes great too! Even after you freeze it.

Serves: 4

Time: 45 Minutes

Ingredients:

- 1 lb. Ground Beef, Lean
- ½ Cup Milk, Low Fat
- 2 Baking Potatoes, Peeled & Diced
- 2 Tablespoons Flour
- 1 Clove Garlic, Minced
- 1 Onion, Chopped
- 4 Cups Mixed Vegetables, Frozen
- 1/2 Cup Cheddar Cheese, Shredded
- ¾ Cup Beef Broth, Reduced Sodium
- Ground Black Pepper to Taste

Directions:

1. Start by dicing your potatoes. Place them in a saucepan and cover them with water. Only use enough water to cover them, and then bring it to a boil.
2. Turn the heat down so that it simmers, covering it and letting it cook for about fifteen minutes. Drain the potatoes, and then mash it. Mix in your milk, and set it to the side.
3. Start by heating the oven to 375.
4. Brown your meat, garlic and onion in a skillet, and then stir in your flour. Cook it for a full minute, and make sure that you stir it constantly. Pour your broth in, and then cook it until it becomes thick and starts to bubble. Stir occasionally during this time.

5. Spoon your mixture into an eight inch dish, and spread your mashed potatoes over your meat and vegetable mixture. Sprinkle the cheese over it.

6. Bake it for twenty-five minutes. It should be hot and bubbly.

46. Taco Soup

Soups are a great meal prepping food because they're filling and keep in the freezer for a long time. You can freeze most soups for about three months.

Serves: 4

Time: 40 Minutes

Ingredients:

- 1 lb. Ground Bee
- 16 Ounces Corn, Canned & Drained
- 1 Brown Onion, Chopped
- 16 Ounces Black Beans, Canned & Drained
- 14 Ounces Tomato Sauce, Canned
- 28 Ounces Tomatoes, Crushed & Canned
- 2 Green Chilies, Diced
- Cilantro for Garnish
- Tortilla Chips for Serving

Directions:

1. Start by browning your meat over medium-high heat, and then add in your onions. Cook until your onions are translucent, and then drain the excess liquid off.
2. Stir your taco seasoning in, and then add in your tomatoes, tomato sauce, black beans, corn, and green chili. Reduce the heat to a simmer, and then cook for about twenty-five minutes.
3. Serve with tortilla chips and cilantro when you're ready to serve. Portion it out, and allow it to cool before freezing it.

47. Zucchini Lasagna

Noodles may not freeze well, but vegetables do, making this a great meal prepping dinner recipe. The best part is that you don't need side dishes with it, but garlic bread does go well.

Serves: 6

Time: 45 Minutes

Ingredients:

- 1 Tablespoon Olive Oil
- 2 Onions, Sliced Thin
- 4 Tomatoes, Sliced ¼ Inch Thick
- 2 Zucchinis, Large & Sliced ¼ Inch Thick
- 6-8 Basil Leaves, Fresh & Chopped
- 8 Ounces Mozzarella, Shredded
- Ground Black Pepper to Taste

Directions:

1. Start by greasing a casserole dish using your olive oil.
2. Place your zucchini in a layer on the bottom, and then spread a layer of tomatoes on top of your zucchini. Place a layer of onion on top of your tomato, and then top with half of your basil before seasoning it with your pepper. Sprinkle a layer of shredded cheese on top. Make sure that you only use about half of your cheese, and then keep layering your vegetables and cheese until there isn't anything left.
3. Allow your oven to heat to 400 degrees, and then cook your lasagna for a half hour.
4. Allow it to cool before freezing.

48. Chicken Fried Rice

If you're low on time, then try this chicken fried rice as a one dish meal that you can freeze.

Serves: 6

Time: 35 Minutes

Ingredients:

- ½ Tablespoon Sesame Oil
- 6 Cups Rice, Cooked
- 3 Cups Mixed Vegetables, Frozen
- 1 lb. Chicken, Cooked & Cubed
- 5 Eggs, Beaten
- 1/3 Cup Soy Sauce
- Black Pepper to Taste
- Vegetable Oil as Needed

Directions:

1. Start by heating your oil in a skillet, scrambling your eggs. Set your now scrambled eggs to the side
2. Add in your sesame oil to the same pan, and toss in your chicken. Cook for about four minutes.
3. Next, stir in your soy sauce and mixed vegetables. You'll want to cook until your vegetables are tender, and then season with black pepper.
4. Mix everything together, and allow it to cool before portioning it out to freeze.

49. Mushroom Pasta Sauce

Pasta is supposed to be an easy meal, but if you don't like jarred sauce, then it can be hard and time consuming. That's where a healthy creamy sauce like this comes in handy. You can just heat up your sauce in the microwave and cook your pasta or serve it over zucchini noodles.

Serves: 4

Time: 20 Minutes

Ingredients:

- 8 Cloves Garlic, Chopped Fine
- 2 Tablespoons Olive Oil
- 5 Cups Mushrooms, Chopped
- 1 Sprig Rosemary, Fresh & Chopped Fine
- ½ Cup Sour Cream
- 3 Ounces White Wine
- ½ Cup Yogurt, Plain

Directions:

1. Start by drizzling your oil in a pan, turning the heat to medium.
2. Add in your rosemary, mushrooms and garlic. Mix well and sauté until your mushrooms start to become colored and shrink some
3. Add in your winner, allowing it to simmer until your alcohol evaporates.
4. Once your alcohol has evaporated, then add in your yogurt and sour cream. Stir well.
5. Turn off the heat, and then divide it between four containers. Seal once it's cooled, and then freeze until you're ready to use it.

50. Broccoli Soup

This is another soup that you can keep in your freezer for up to three months, and it's healthy and easy to make.

Serves: 4

Time: 30 Minutes

Ingredients:

- 4 Cups Chicken Stock
- 1 Carrot, Chopped & Peeled
- 2 Cloves Garlic, Minced
- 4 Tablespoons Butter
- 1 ½ lbs. Broccoli Florets
- 3 Tablespoons All Purpose Flour
- ½ Cup Cream
- 1 Brown Onion, Diced
- Sea Salt & Black Pepper to Taste

Directions:

1. Melt your butter in a pot, using medium-high heat. Add in your onion, carrot and broccoli. Sauté until your onions turn slightly translucent, which should take about five minutes.
2. Season with sea salt and black pepper before adding in your garlic and flour. Cook for another minute before adding your stock and allowing it to come to a boil.
3. Simmer for about fifteen minutes. Your broccoli should become tender, and then add in your cream. Use an immersion blender to puree the soup, and then serve hot with bread.
4. Allow it to cool, and then freeze it for up to three months.

51. Lamb Curry

This lamb curry is made with couscous, and so it's packed full of protein and fiber to keep you full through the night.

Serves: 6

Time: 30 Minutes

Ingredients:

- Olive Oil as Needed
- 2 Onions, Chopped Roughly
- 1 Teaspoon Ground Turmeric
- 1 Teaspoon Chili Powder
- 1 Teaspoon Coriander, Dried
- 1 Teaspoon Cumin, Dried
- ½ Teaspoon Cinnamon
- 20 Ounces Lamb Steak, Cubed
- 28 Ounces Tomatoes, Canned & Chopped
- 2 Cups Lamb Stock
- 2 Cups Couscous, Dried
- Sea Salt & Black Pepper to Taste

Directions:

1. Start by drizzling your pan with olive oil, using medium heat.
2. Add in your chili powder, cumin, onions, turmeric, cinnamon and coriander. Cook until your onions are soft.
3. Add your lamb cubes in, stirring until they're coated with spices. Brown your meat, which should take three to five minutes
4. Add your tomatoes, sea salt, and black pepper and lamb stock. Make sure to mix well.
5. Put your lid on the pot, and then simmer it for twenty-five minutes on low heat. Your sauce should begin to thicken.

6. Now while your curry is cooking, you need to prepare the couscous. To do this place your dried couscous in a bowl. Bring two and a half cups of water to a boil, and then pour it over your couscous. Let it sit for five minutes while covered.

7. Uncover your couscous, adding sea salt and pepper before fluffing.

8. Divide it between your six containers, and then allow your curry to cool before dividing it between your containers as well.

9. Freeze until needed.

52.Cranberry Pork Chops

Pork chops are able to be frozen, but remember that the quality of your pork will make a large difference in the quality once it's thawed too.

Serves: 4

Time: 8 Hours 10 Minutes

Ingredients:

- Sea Salt & Black Pepper to Taste
- 4 Pork Chops, Boneless
- 1 Onion, Chopped
- 2 Tablespoons Butter, Chopped
- 1 Celery Stalk, Chopped
- 2 Cloves Garlic, Minced
- 1 Cup Cranberries, Fresh
- ½ Teaspoon Thyme, Dried
- ¼ Cup Chicken Broth
- 2 Tablespoons Brown Sugar

Directions:

1. Start by melting your butter over medium heat in a large skillet before adding in your onion, sea salt, garlic and celery. Cook while stirring until your vegetables become tender.
2. Place your vegetables, pork chops, pepper, cranberries, brown sugar and thyme in a slow cooker.
3. Pour in your broth, cooking on low for six to eight hours. The pork chops should be cooked all the way through.
4. Allow your pork chops and sauce to cool completely before you portion them out and freeze them.

53. Chicken with Broccoli

No need to get take out when you have this great chicken and broccoli recipe! Just serve it over rice.

Serves: 4

Time: 35 Minutes

Ingredients:

- 2 Cups Broccoli Florets
- 1 lb. Chicken Breasts, Sliced
- 1 Inch Piece Ginger, Peeled & Chopped
- 1 Red Bell Pepper, Seeded & Sliced
- 4 Teaspoons Soy Sauce
- 1 Tablespoon Honey, Raw
- 1 Tablespoon Rice Wine Vinegar
- 2 Scallions, Fresh & Diced
- 2 Cloves Garlic, Chopped
- 1 Carrot, Julienned
- Sesame Oil as Needed
- Vegetable Oil as Needed
- 2 Cups Rice, Cooked

Directions:

1. Start by whisking your rice wine vinegar, soy sauce and honey together. Make sure it's mixed well.
2. Heat the vegetable oil over high heat in your wok, and then add half of your garlic, scallion and ginger with your chicken into the pan. Fry for about two minutes. Your chicken should start to brown.
3. Pour in your soy sauce mixture, and then simmer until your chicken glazes. Set it to the side.
4. Place your pan over high heat again, swirling in more of your vegetable oil, adding in the rest of your garlic, scallion and ginger. Add

in your bell peppers, carrot and broccoli. Fry for one to two minutes before adding in a third a cup of water.

5. Cover your wok, allowing your vegetables to steam until they are tender but crisp. This should take about five minutes.

6. Uncover your pan, adding in the rest of your soy sauce mixture, and then cook for another one to two minutes.

7. Add your chicken back in, and stir to combine. Drizzle lightly with sesame oil.

8. Divide your rice between your containers, and then top with your stir fry.

9. Allow to cool before freezing.

54. Tikka Masala

This dish is traditionally made with chicken, and it's easy to freeze and makes a large quantity. It's perfect to help stock your freezer.

Serves: 10

Time: 40 Minutes

Ingredients:

- 8 Chicken Breasts, Cubed
- 4 Tablespoons Tomato Puree
- ½ Cup Tikka Masala Paste
- 4 Onions, Diced
- 4 Tablespoons Vegetable Oil
- 1 ½ Tablespoons Butter
- 2 Red Peppers, Seeded & Diced
- 28 Ounces Tomatoes, Canned & Chopped
- 2 Tablespoons Mango Chutney
- ½ Cup Yogurt, Plain
- ½ Cup Double Cream
- Sea Salt & Black Pepper to Taste
- Fresh Coriander to Garnish if Desired

Directions:

1. Start by heating your butter and oil together in a pan, adding in your onion. Season it with salt, and cook on low heat for five minutes. Your onions should become soft.
2. Add in your tikka masala paste and peppers, cooking for another five minutes.
3. Add in your chicken, stirring to coat and cooking for another two minutes.

4. Pour in your tomatoes, add your puree, and add 2/3 cup of water. Cover, allowing it to simmer for fifteen minutes. You'll need to stir occasionally. Your chicken should be cooked all the way through.

5. Remove it from heat, adding in your cream, yogurt and mango chutney. Stir gently, and then garnish with coriander if desired.

6. Allow to cool completely before freezing.

55. Green Potato Curry

Curry is filling and easy to heat up, and it can be kept in the fridge or freezer. Just microwave it for a few minutes, and stir to make sure it's heated all the way through when you're ready to eat it.

Serves: 6

Time: 30 Minutes

Ingredients:

- Olive Oil to Taste
- 1 Onion, Chopped Fine
- 4 Cloves Garlic, Chopped Fine
- 5 Potatoes, Cubed
- 4 Tablespoons Green Curry Paste
- 2 Cups Peas, Frozen
- 2 Cups Green Beans, Frozen
- 1 Cup Vegetable Broth
- 3 Cups Coconut Milk
- Sea Salt to Taste

Directions:

1. Drizzle your olive oil into a pan, and then put it over medium heat. Add in your curry paste, garlic and onion, stirring. Sauté for a few minutes. Your curry should become fragrant.
2. Add your beans, peas, potatoes, and broth in. stir well, and then add in your coconut milk, stirring again. Season with a pinch of salt.
3. Allow it to come to a boil, allowing it to boil for twenty minutes. Your potatoes should be soft.
4. Let it cool before dividing it up to freeze.

56. Beef & Vegetable Meatloaf

If you're already missing traditional meals, then this meatloaf is for you. It heats well once it's sliced, and you can serve it with just about any vegetable or potato dish on the side. Store it either in the fridge or freezer.

Serves: 4

Time: 1 Hour 15 Minutes

Ingredients:

- 1 lb. Ground Beef
- 1 Onion, Diced
- 1 Carrot, Grated
- 1 Cup Brown Rice, Cooked
- 1 Zucchini, Grated
- 1 Egg, Beaten
- 1 Tablespoon Tamari
- ¾ Cup Greek Yogurt, Plain
- 2 Tablespoons Parsley, Fresh & Chopped
- 1 Teaspoon Ground Black Pepper

Directions:

1. Start by heating your oven to 360, and then grease a loaf pan.
2. In a bowl, combine all ingredients, mixing them well.
3. Place the mixture in your pan, baking for an hour.
4. Let it stand for ten minutes before portioning it out to freeze it. Make sure it's cooled down before you freeze it!

57. Mushroom & Chicken Pie

If you're looking for a dinner with very little time, then this might be for you! You can serve it with sides or have it on the go.

Serves: 6

Time: 1 Hour

Ingredients:

- 2 Chicken Breasts, Sliced
- 2 Cups Mushrooms, Sliced Thin
- 1 Leek, Diced
- 3 Bacon Rashers, Diced
- 1 Tablespoon Olive Oil
- 1 Teaspoon Smoked Paprika
- 1 Cup Cheese, Grated
- ¼ Cup Flour, Plain
- 1 Cup Peas, Frozen
- ½ Cup Vegetable Stock
- 4 Sheets Short crust Pastry, Frozen
- 1 Tablespoon Butter

Directions:

1. Start by heating your oven to 390, and then grease a six hole muffin tin. Cut your pasty to line each tin, and then bake for eight to ten minutes. Your pasty should become browned.
2. In a bowl, add your chicken and coat it in your flour and smoked paprika.
3. Heat your oil over medium heat in a pan, adding in your bacon and leek. Allow it to cook for about three minutes.
4. Add in your coated chicken, and then brown for another three minutes.

5. Add in your peas, stock and mushrooms, and then bring the mixture to a boil. Reduce the heat to low, allowing it to simmer for ten minutes. Your sauce should thicken, and then allow it to cool.

6. Spoon the filling in your pasty case, sprinkling cheese over it.

7. Place your tin back in the oven, cooking for another twenty to twenty-five minutes more. Your pastry should become golden.

8. Allow to cool before freezing.

Two Week Meal Plan

You may be wondering how to schedule everything in, which is where this chapter will help. Here is a look at your first two weeks meal prepping. For the sake of an example, you'll meal prep on Sunday, which is when the majority of people have the most time.

Before Week 1: Your Sunday

Meals:

- Berry Chia Pots
- Banana Pancakes
- Fajita Bowls
- Salmon with Greens (Remember that when you make this meal you'll want to keep your greens separate in the fridge until you're ready to eat so that you can freeze your salmon!)
- Chia & Maple Chickpeas
- Apple Pie Balls
- Easy Shepherd's Pie
- Lamb Curry
- Chicken & Broccoli

Time Cooking: 4 hours 40 Minutes

Week 1: Monday

Breakfast: Berry Chia Pots

Lunch: Stuffed Sweet Potato

Dinner: Easy Shepherd's Pie

Snacks: Either Apple Pie Balls or Chia & Maple Chickpeas

Week 1: Tuesday

Breakfast: Berry Chia Pots

Lunch: Salmon with Greens

Dinner: Lamb Curry

Snacks: Either Apple Pie Balls or Chia & Maple Chickpeas

Week 1: Wednesday

Breakfast: Banana Pancakes

Lunch: Stuffed Sweet Potato

Dinner: Chicken & Broccoli

Snacks: Either Apple Pie Balls or Chia & Maple Chickpeas

Week 1: Thursday

Breakfast: Berry Chia Pots

Lunch: Salmon with Greens

Dinner: Lamb & Curry

Snacks: Either Apple Pie Balls or Chia & Maple Chickpeas

Week 1: Friday

Breakfast: Banana Pancakes

Lunch: Fajita Bowl

Dinner: Easy Shepherd's Pie

Snacks: Either Apple Pie Balls or Chia & Maple Chickpeas

Week 1: Saturday

Breakfast: Berry Chia Pots

Lunch: Stuffed Sweet Potato

Dinner: Chicken & Broccoli

Snacks: Either Apple Pie Balls or Chia & Maple Chickpeas

Week 1: Sunday

You shouldn't have to prep for your week and still cook for the day!

Breakfast: Banana Pancakes

Lunch: Salmon with Greens

Dinner: Lamb Curry

Snacks: Either Apple Pie Balls or Chia & Maple Chickpeas

What's Left In Your Freezer

You may have found that week to be a little bit repetitive, but you're slowly building up your freezer. Here's what you should have left in your freezer if you're feeding one person.

- 1 Serving Banana Pancakes
- 1 Serving Stuffed Sweet Potatoes
- 1 Serving Salmon with Greens
- 3 Servings Fajita Bowls
- 2 Servings Chicken and Broccoli
- 1 Serving Lamb Curry
- 1 Serving Easy Shepherd's Pie

Now that you have these, your next week will have a little more variation in it. To make sure that nothing goes bad in the freezer, remember to mark the day you mark down the day you should throw it away. This will help you to organize your meals later on. You'll also have whatever snacks are left in your freezer to get you through the next week.

Starting Week 2: Sunday

You already know what you're eating on this day since it was listed in last week's meal plan, but here is what you should cook and how long it will take you.

Meals:

- Green Smoothie Packets
- Breakfast Burritos
- Tropical Smoothie Packets
- Roasted Vegetable Salad
- Smoked Salmon Wraps
- Chocolate Energy Balls
- Apricot Energy Bars
- Broccoli Soup
- Green Potato Curry
- Beef & Vegetable Meat Loaf

Time Cooking: 4 Hours

Week 2: Monday

Breakfast: Green Smoothie Packet
Lunch: Roasted Vegetable Salad
Dinner: Broccoli Soup
Snacks: Chia & Maple Chickpeas, Apple Pie Balls, Chocolate Energy Balls, or Apricot Energy Bars

Week 2: Tuesday

Breakfast: Breakfast Burritos
Lunch: Smoked Salmon Wraps
Dinner: Green Potato Curry
Snacks: Chia & Maple Chickpeas, Apple Pie Balls, Chocolate Energy Balls, or Apricot Energy Bars

Week 2: Wednesday

Breakfast: Banana Pancakes

Lunch: Roasted Vegetable Salad

Dinner: Chicken & Broccoli

Snacks: Chia & Maple Chickpeas, Apple Pie Balls, Chocolate Energy Balls, or Apricot Energy Bars

Week 2: Thursday

Breakfast: Breakfast Burritos

Lunch: Salmon with Greens

Dinner: Beef & Vegetable Meat Loaf

Snacks: Chia & Maple Chickpeas, Apple Pie Balls, Chocolate Energy Balls, or Apricot Energy Bars

Week 2: Friday

Breakfast: Tropical Smoothie Packet

Lunch: Fajita Bowl

Dinner: Green Potato Curry

Snacks: Chia & Maple Chickpeas, Apple Pie Balls, Chocolate Energy Balls, or Apricot Energy Bars

Week 2: Saturday

Breakfast: Breakfast Burrito

Lunch: Smoked Salmon Wraps

Dinner: Broccoli Soup

Snacks: Chia & Maple Chickpeas, Apple Pie Balls, Chocolate Energy Balls, or Apricot Energy Bars

Week 2: Sunday

Remember that there is no reason to cook on a day that you're setting aside to meal prep!

Breakfast: Tropical Smoothie Packet

Lunch: Fajita Bowl

Dinner: Green Potato Curry

Snacks: Chia & Maple Chickpeas, Apple Pie Balls, Chocolate Energy Balls, or Apricot Energy Bars

What's Left in Your Freezer

Now you'll see that in week two you had a lot more variety, and while you depleted some of your stash you still have a variety in your freezer. Dedicate another few hours on Sunday for week three, but keep in mind the food that might be going bad in the next week or two. Here is what should be left in your freezer.

- 6 Green Smoothie Packets
- 21 Breakfast Burritos
- 5 Tropical Smoothie Packets
- 2 Servings Roasted Vegetable Salad
- 2 Smoked Salmon Wraps
- 2 Servings Broccoli Soup
- 4 Servings Green Potato Curry
- 3 Servings Beef & Vegetable Meatloaf
- 1 Stuffed Sweet Potato
- 1 Fajita Bowl
- 1 Serving Chicken & Broccoli
- 1 Serving Lamb Curry
- 1 Serving Easy Shepherd's Pie

You'll also have whatever snacks that you didn't eat!

Conclusion

Now you know everything you need to get started with meal prepping to make your life easier and eat healthier! There's no reason to worry about your first two weeks with the two week meal plan included in this book. Meal prepping doesn't have to be hard, especially if you have all of your ingredients. Just remember that lists will be your best friend when cooking and shopping. Organization makes meal prepping much easier, since you won't waste time looking for ingredients, going on second shopping trips, or trying to figure out what to do first. Meal prepping is meant to make your life easier. When most people spend hours a day cooking, you'll spend only a few hours each week, leaving more time to do what you want.